Healthy teeth healthy me....

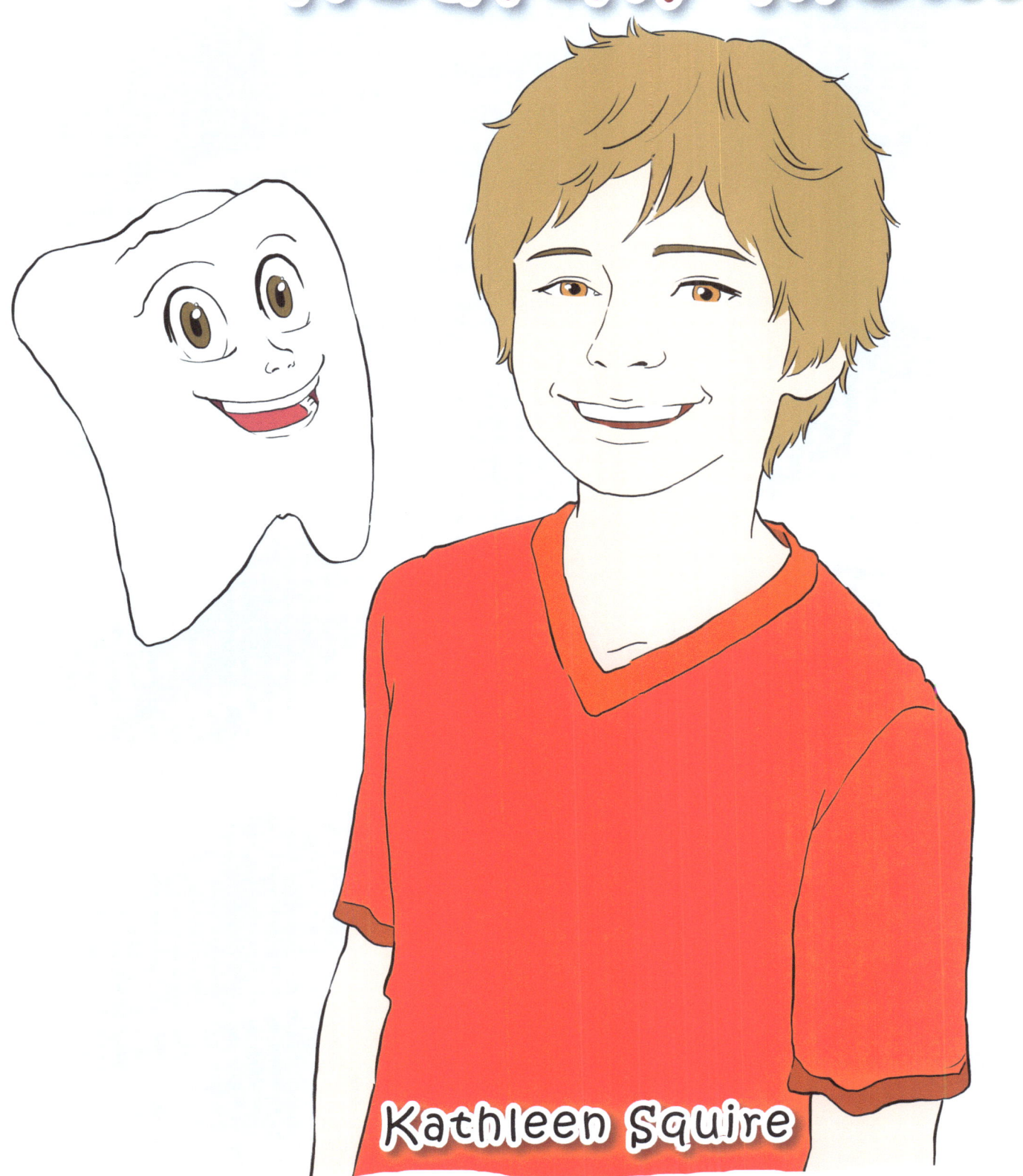

Kathleen Squire

Order this book online at www.trafford.com
or email orders@trafford.com

Most Trafford titles are also available at major online book retailers.

Printed in the United States of America.

ISBN: 978-1-4669-9093-7 (sc)
        978-1-4669-9092-0 (e)

Library of Congress Control Number: 2013907349

Our mission is to efficiently provide the world's finest, most comprehensive book publishing service, enabling every author to experience success. To find out how to publish your book, your way, and have it available worldwide, visit us online at www.trafford.com

Trafford rev. 04/22/2013

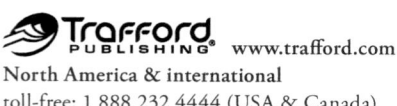 www.trafford.com

North America & international
toll-free: 1 888 232 4444 (USA & Canada)
phone: 250 383 6864 ♦ fax: 812 355 4082

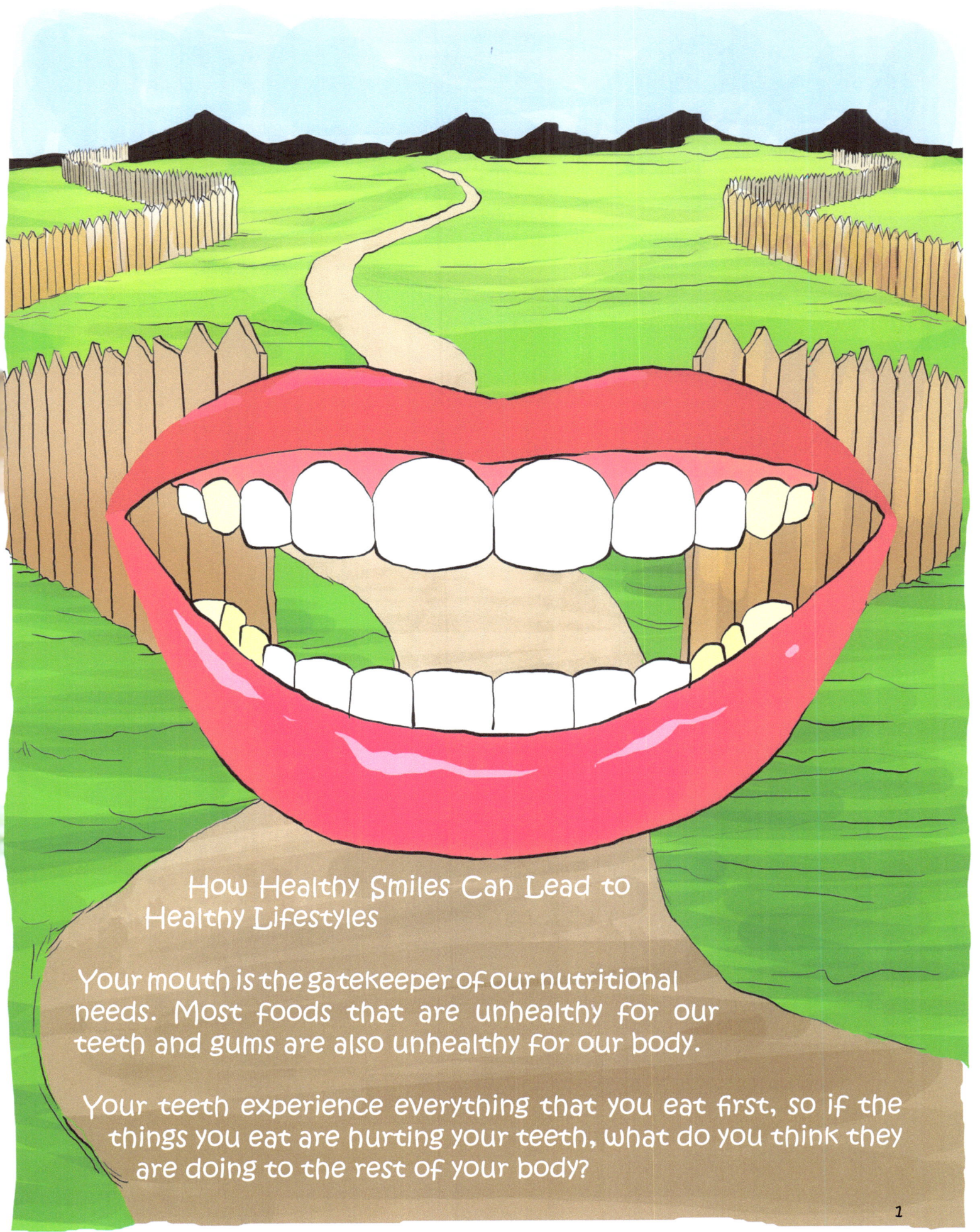

How Healthy Smiles Can Lead to Healthy Lifestyles

Your mouth is the gatekeeper of our nutritional needs. Most foods that are unhealthy for our teeth and gums are also unhealthy for our body.

Your teeth experience everything that you eat first, so if the things you eat are hurting your teeth, what do you think they are doing to the rest of your body?

As a dental professional, it is part of my job to educate patients about proper home care and nutrition to care for their teeth to last a lifetime.

Taking care of your mouth is equally important as taking care of your body.

Just like washing your hands often helps you from getting sick, brushing and flossing daily prevent tooth decay and gum disease.

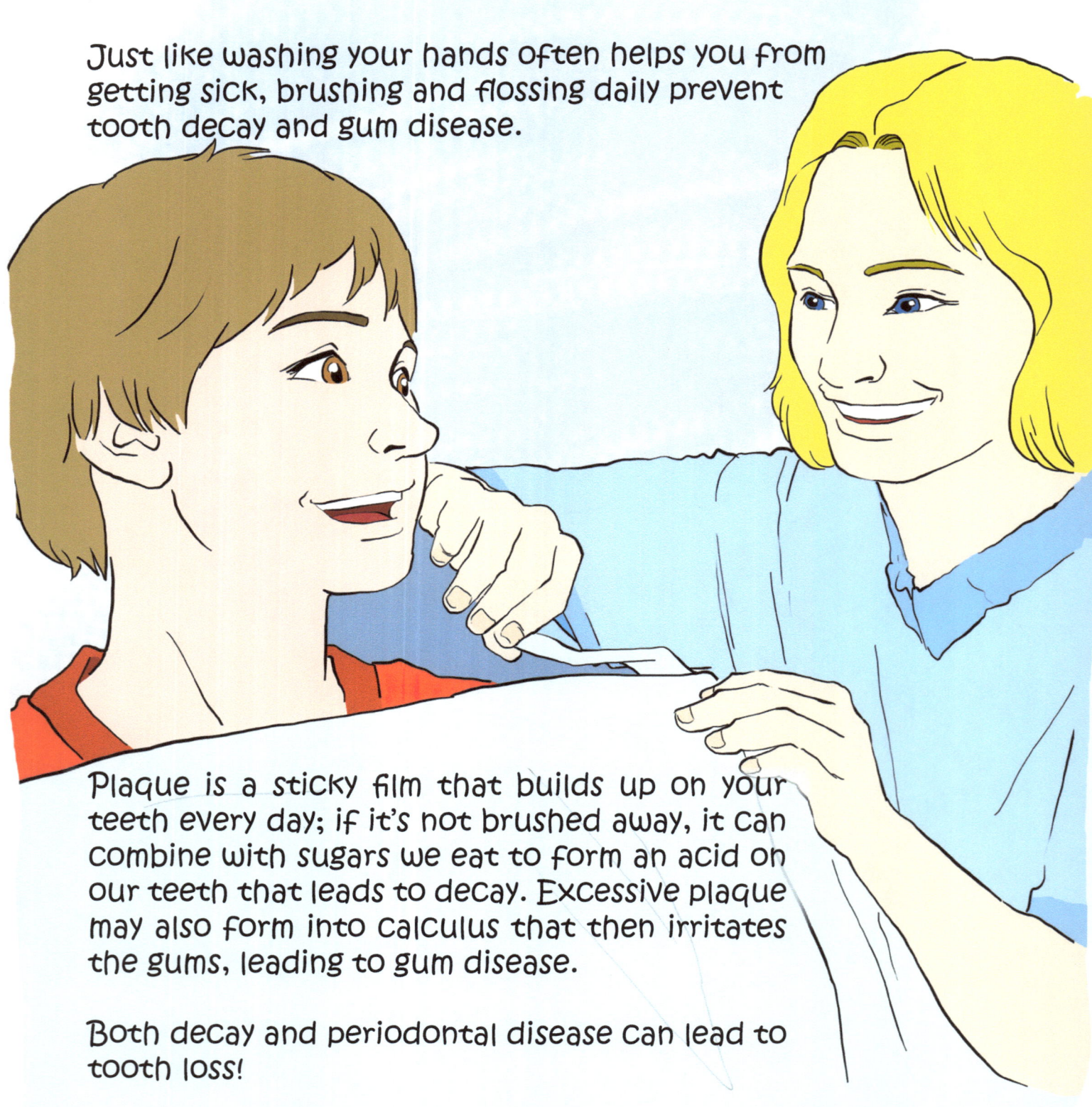

Plaque is a sticky film that builds up on your teeth every day; if it's not brushed away, it can combine with sugars we eat to form an acid on our teeth that leads to decay. Excessive plaque may also form into calculus that then irritates the gums, leading to gum disease.

Both decay and periodontal disease can lead to tooth loss!

Are your teeth important to you?

Think about how often you use your teeth each day.

Eating breakfast, lunch, and dinner.

Speaking to our friends and family.

Smiling—did you ever notice that if you smile at someone, they almost always smile back? Smiling is contagious!

Would you smile as much
If you were missing some teeth?
Would it be harder to make sounds when you speak?
What kinds of foods would you be able to eat
If you were missing too many teeth?

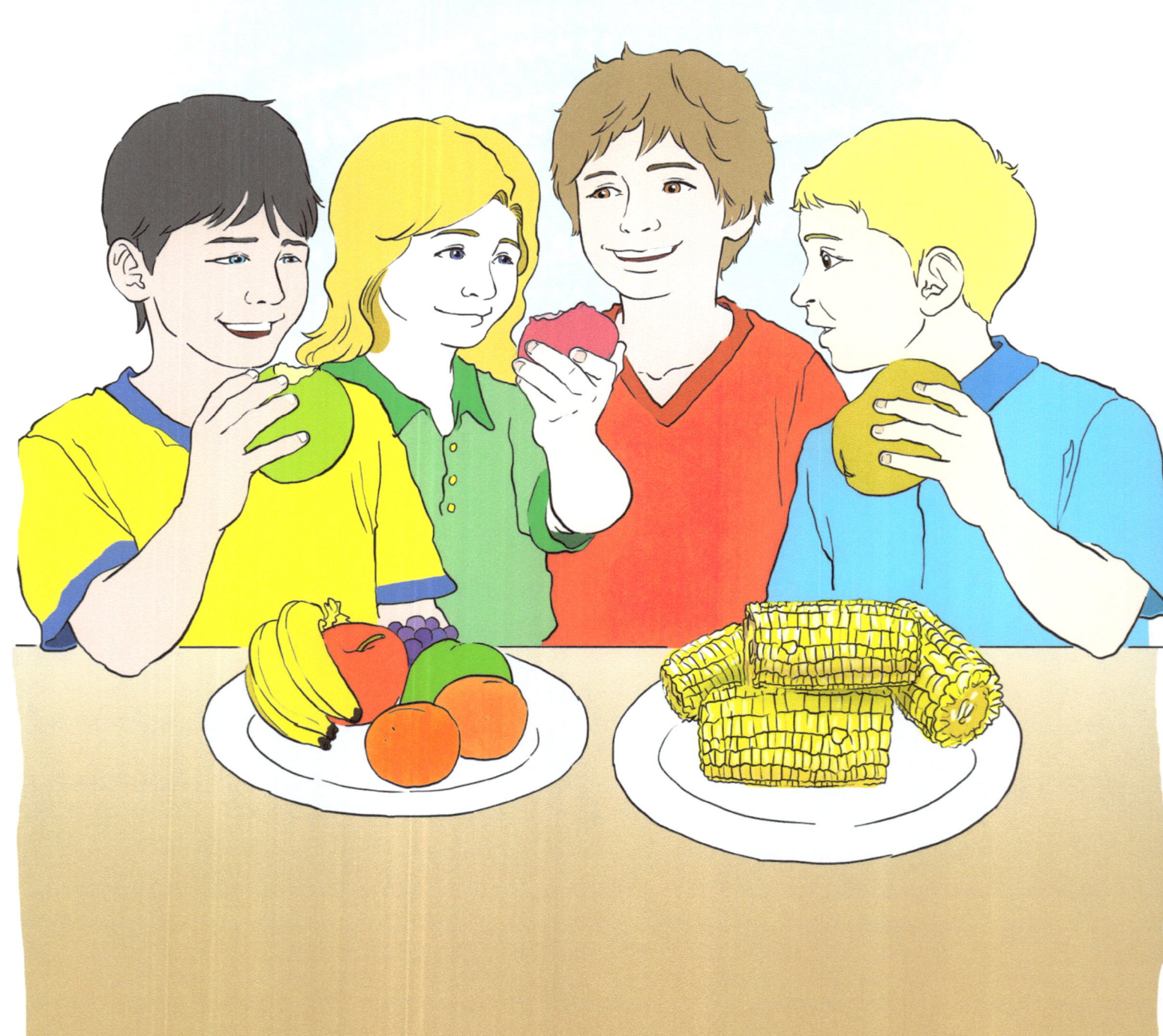

This book is designed to encourage you to make healthy choices that will not only help you have a healthy mouth but, in doing so, will also benefit your body!

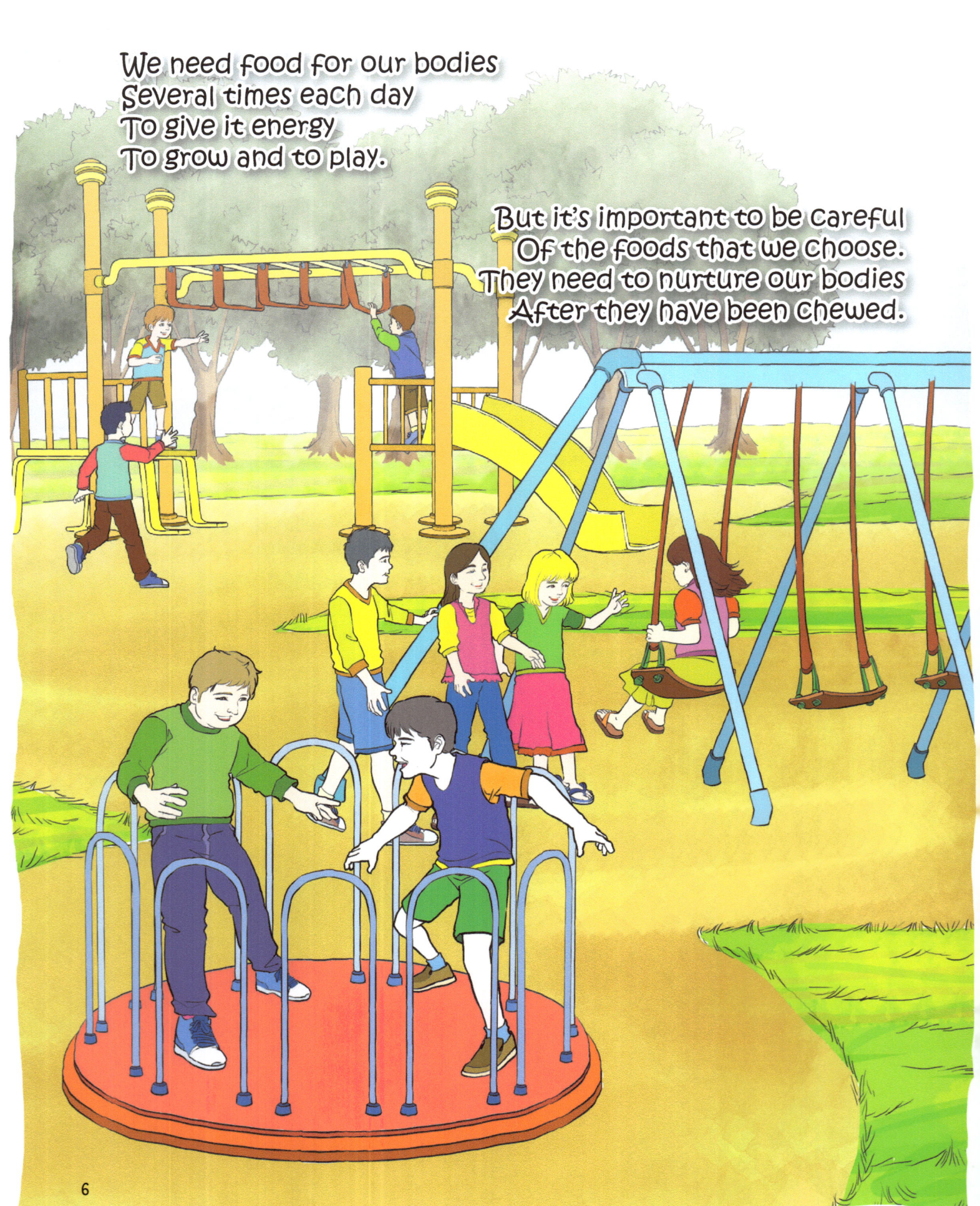

We need food for our bodies
Several times each day
To give it energy
To grow and to play.

But it's important to be careful
Of the foods that we choose.
They need to nurture our bodies
After they have been chewed.

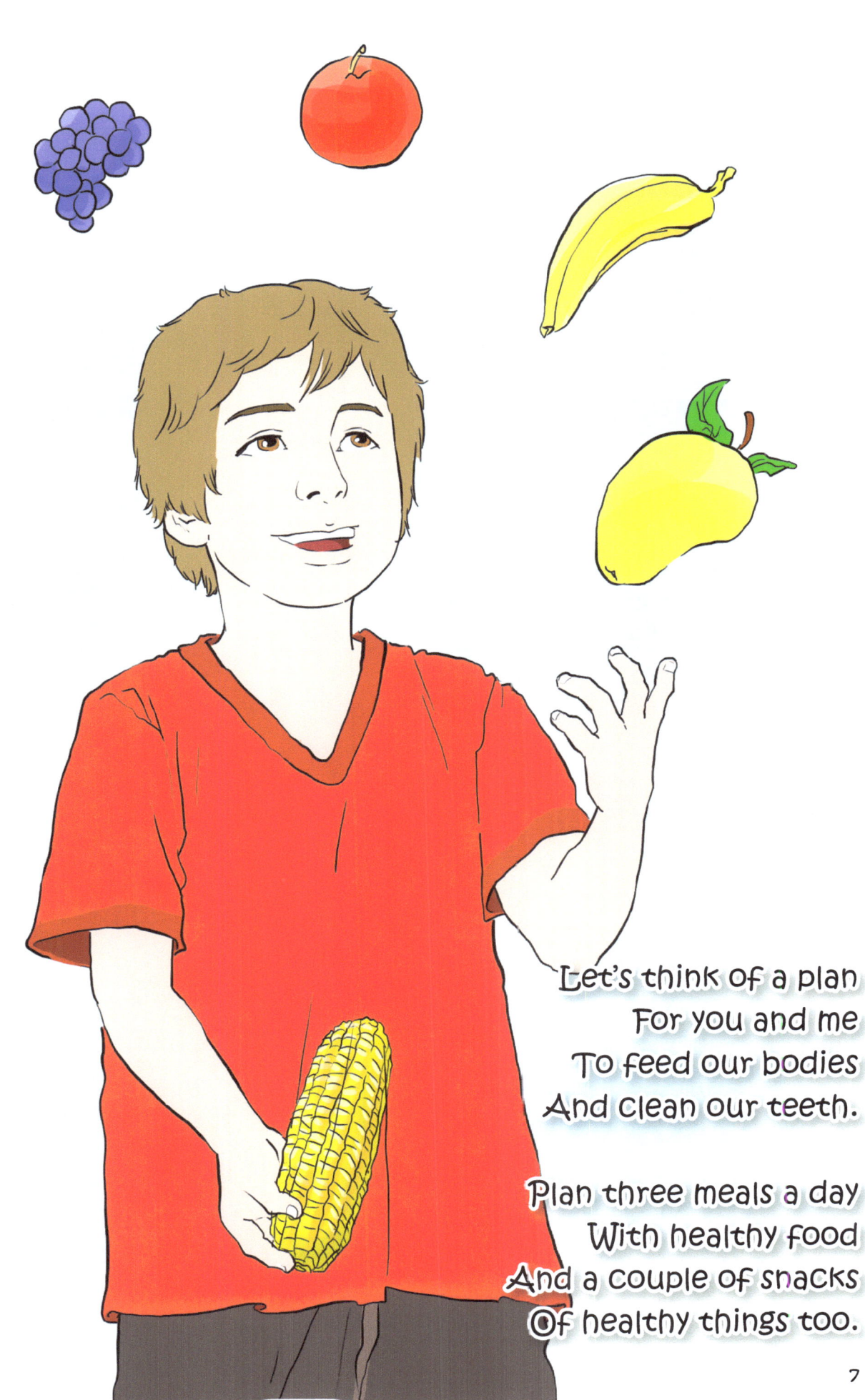

Let's think of a plan
For you and me
To feed our bodies
And clean our teeth.

Plan three meals a day
With healthy food
And a couple of snacks
Of healthy things too.

7

Be sure not to snack throughout the day.
There is a word for that; it is called graze.

Grazing is something that cows can do.
They munch on grass the whole day through.

The grass does not cause tooth decay.
That is why they can do it every day.

But when people graze, they do not eat grass.
They tend to eat a crunchy food snack.
These are the types that stick to your teeth.
When mixed with plaque, they'll form a cavity!

Also beware of sipping on drinks all day
As they coat your teeth and cause decay.
If you must sip, choose H_2O.
There is nothing harmful in that, you know.

Let's determine what we can eat.
We have meals and snacks
And occasional treats.
Meals should be healthy,
And snacks should be too.
Treats should be fun
But only a few.
What makes a food healthy
For your teeth
Is something low in sugar and not too sticky.
What makes a food good for your body would be
A food packed with nutrients and low in calories.

How can you tell if a food is good for your teeth?

When you eat some food and chew it up
Take a look in the mirror and see where it stuck!

On the top of your teeth or maybe in between—these are the types of foods
That you have to be sure to clean!

Dried fruits, chips, and breads are carbohydrates we like to eat.
But after they've been chewed, they tend to stick to our teeth.
If they stay behind too long, they turn to sugar and mix with plaque.
Then they form an acid, and then they attack!

They are also high in calories
And are the types of food we like to graze,
And if you get into that habit, it can cause excess weight gain!

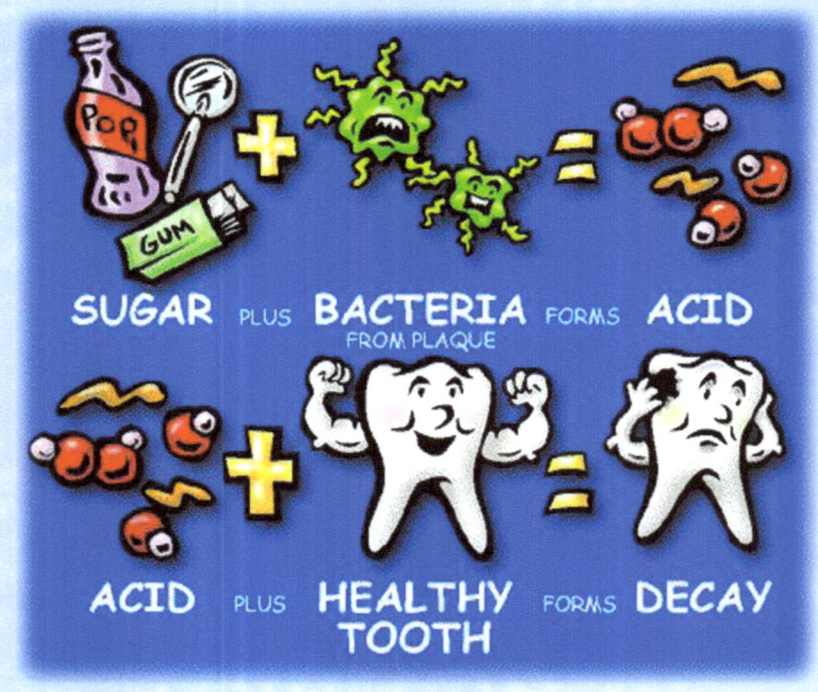

Fruits and veggies are crunchy and sweet,
And they do not naturally harm your teeth.
Nutrient rich and low in calories
That will nurture your body
From your head to your feet.

Proteins are also types of foods that are not cavity prone.
They will help you feel full
And give you muscle tone.

Dairy has protein
And calcium too.
It builds strong teeth
And helps your bones too.

Carbs are things we all like to eat.
You can find them in healthy foods and also in treats,
But beware if they are in sugar form
Because your teeth and your body
Won't be healthy for long.

Let's spend some time evaluating
Some food and drinks.
Before we eat them
We need to think!

In this next section
You will find
Some information
To keep in mind.

The more you know about food you see
Will keep your body and
Teeth healthy!

The colors of the rainbow will form a key
For the things in food
That are good and healthy.

But beware if the storm clouds
As in this key
Are warnings of what may be harmful
For both our bodies and our teeth.

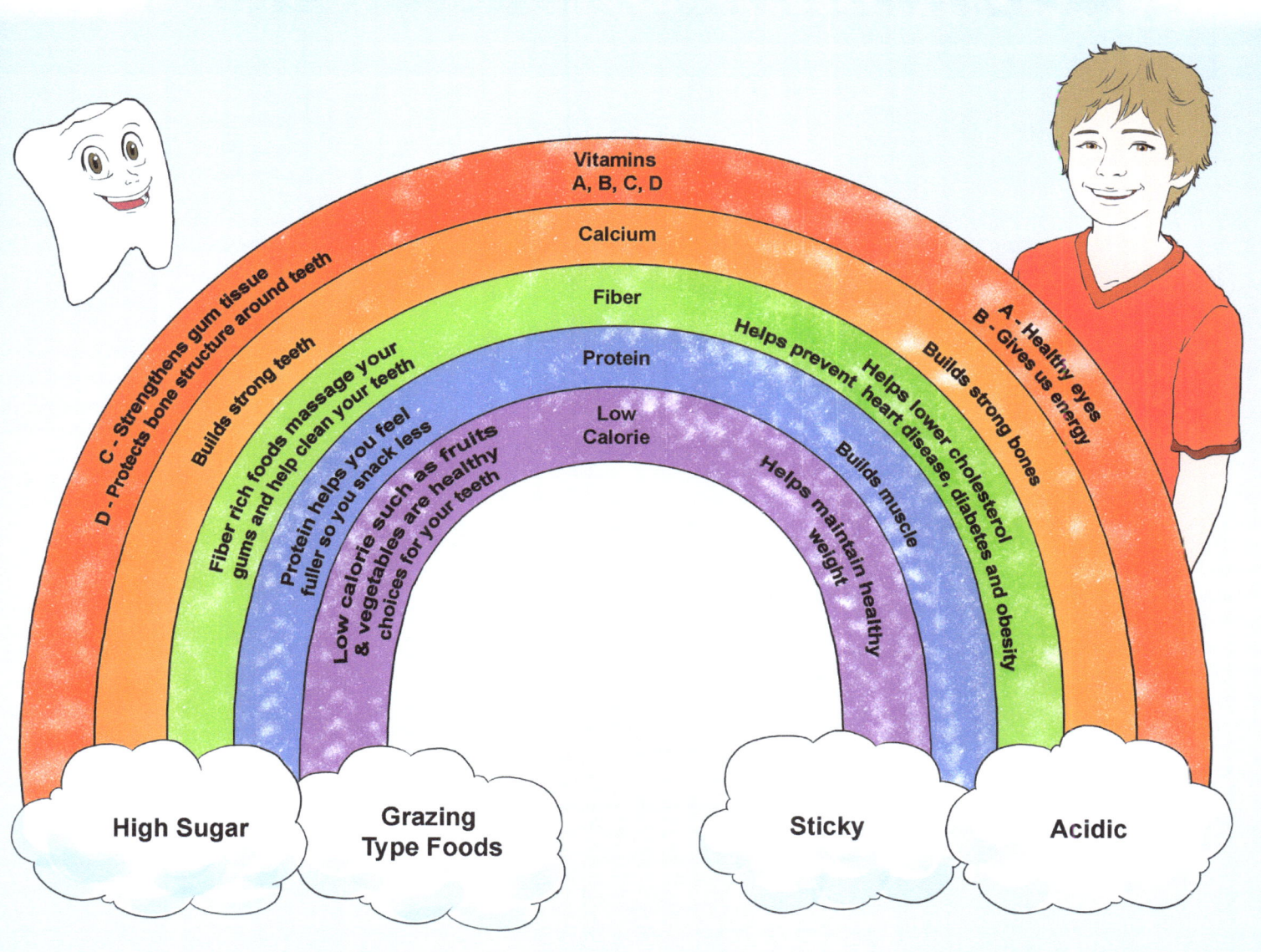

Vitamins
A, B, C, D

Calcium

Fiber

Protein

Low Calorie

A - Healthy eyes
B - Gives us energy

Builds strong bones

Helps lower cholesterol

Helps prevent heart disease, diabetes and obesity

Builds muscle

Helps maintain healthy weight

C - Strengthens gum tissue
D - Protects bone structure around teeth

Builds strong teeth

Fiber rich foods massage your gums and help clean your teeth

Protein helps you feel fuller so you snack less

Low calorie such as fruits & vegetables are healthy choices for your teeth

High Sugar

Grazing Type Foods

Sticky

Acidic

Remember, it's all in moderation
With the foods that we choose.
Eat when you're really hungry or at mealtimes,
Not as reward or to amuse.

Choose foods in their natural state.
Beware of packaged foods.
If they're made to look appealing,
Are they really good for you?

Read on for some food ideas
That have been tried and true.
You'll find that they are tasty
And definitely good for you.

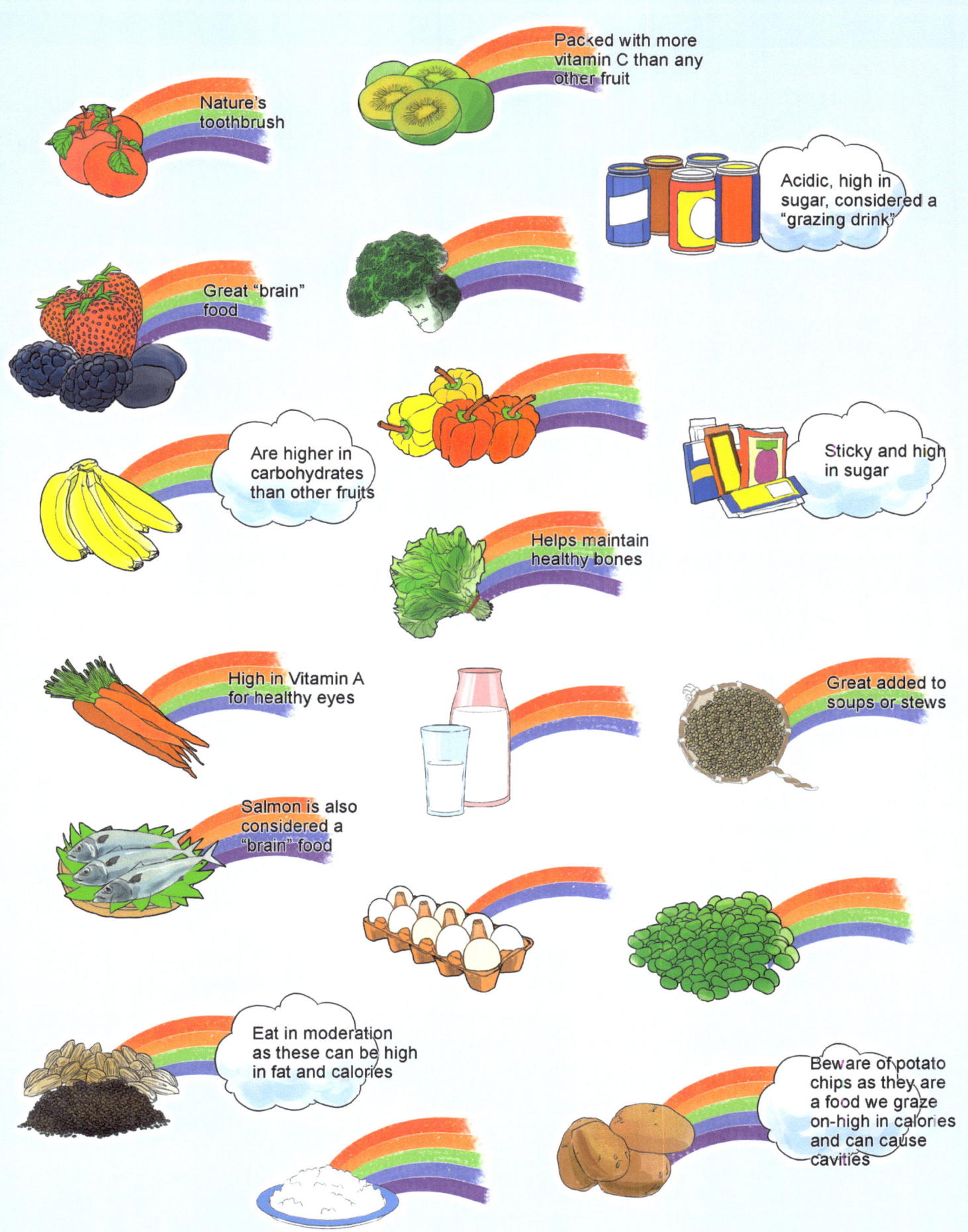

Nature's toothbrush

Packed with more vitamin C than any other fruit

Acidic, high in sugar, considered a "grazing drink"

Great "brain" food

Are higher in carbohydrates than other fruits

Sticky and high in sugar

Helps maintain healthy bones

High in Vitamin A for healthy eyes

Great added to soups or stews

Salmon is also considered a "brain" food

Eat in moderation as these can be high in fat and calories

Beware of potato chips as they are a food we graze on-high in calories and can cause cavities

Trade this

For this

Soda, Juice & Sports Drinks
- Water
- Green Tea
- Fruit smoothie

Something Sweet
- Sliced peppers
- Sliced apples and cinnamon or peanut butter
- Popcorn
- Fill a waffle cone with sliced fruits or berries and yogurt, top with granola

Fruit snacks & Hard Candy
- Frozen berries
- Kale chips
- Jerky
- Whole fruit

Chips, Crackers & Pretzels
- Inside out sandwich-spread mustard on a deli turkey slice, and wrap around a sesame breadstick.
- Put cubes of cheese and grapes on pretzel sticks.
- Popcorn
- Xylitol gum after snacks helps prevent cavities.
- Try whole grain crackers.

Cavities happen when
Sugar and plaque
Mix together to form acid
Then they attack!

Sugars come from many foods that we eat, and they are even in
some foods that do not taste sweet!

Plaque naturally builds up on our teeth every day, and it will
stay there until we brush it away!

Gum disease is something that can make your gums bleed.
It's caused by bacteria in plaque you can't see.
Cleaning your teeth thoroughly is all you can do,
Flossing them once and brushing at least two.

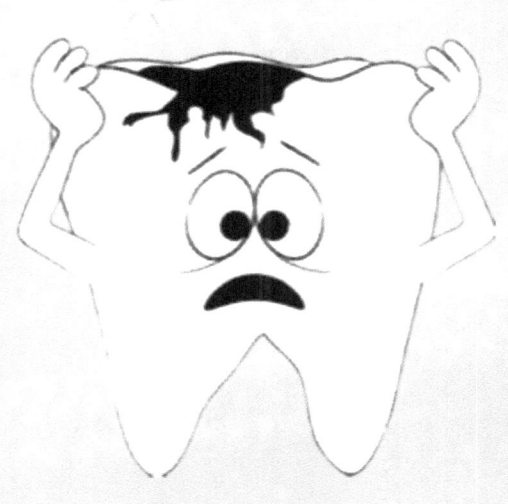

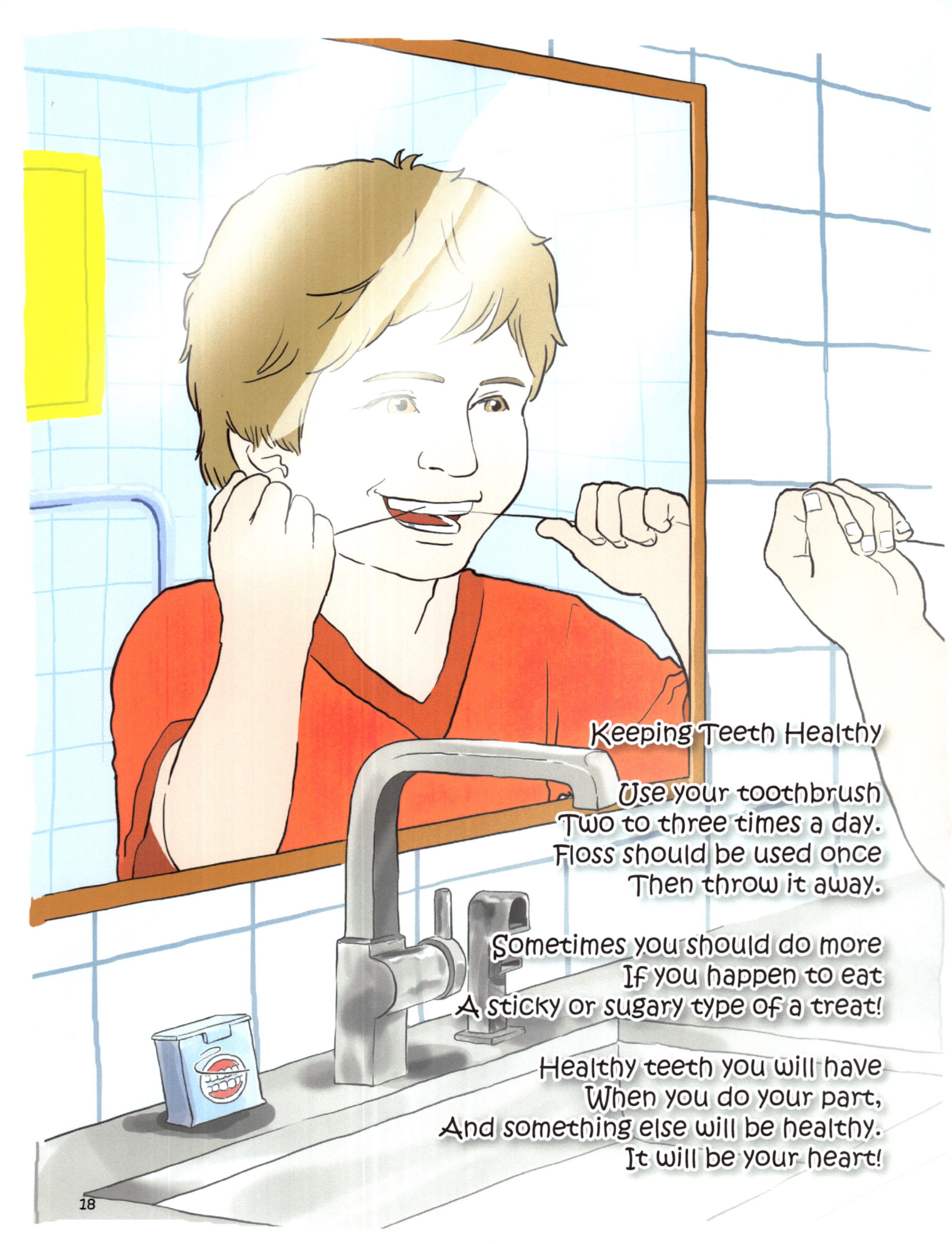

Keeping Teeth Healthy

Use your toothbrush
Two to three times a day.
Floss should be used once
Then throw it away.

Sometimes you should do more
If you happen to eat
A sticky or sugary type of a treat!

Healthy teeth you will have
When you do your part,
And something else will be healthy.
It will be your heart!

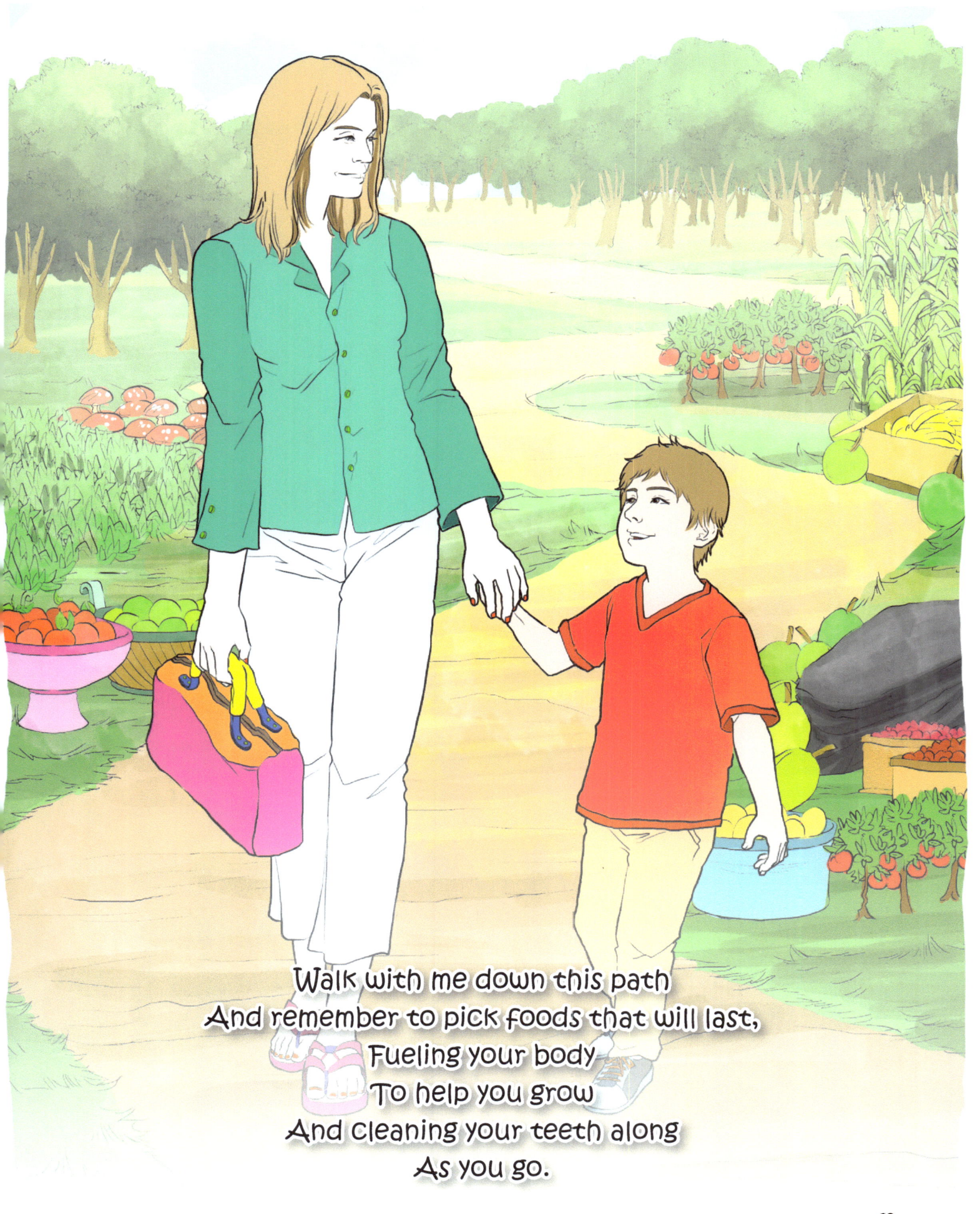

Walk with me down this path
And remember to pick foods that will last,
Fueling your body
To help you grow
And cleaning your teeth along
As you go.

Conclusion

I hope that this book
Taught you a little about
How important it is to take care
Of your mouth.

Remember the gateway
To all that you eat
Is so important.
They are your teeth!

Smile on!